Title: Nurturing the Future:

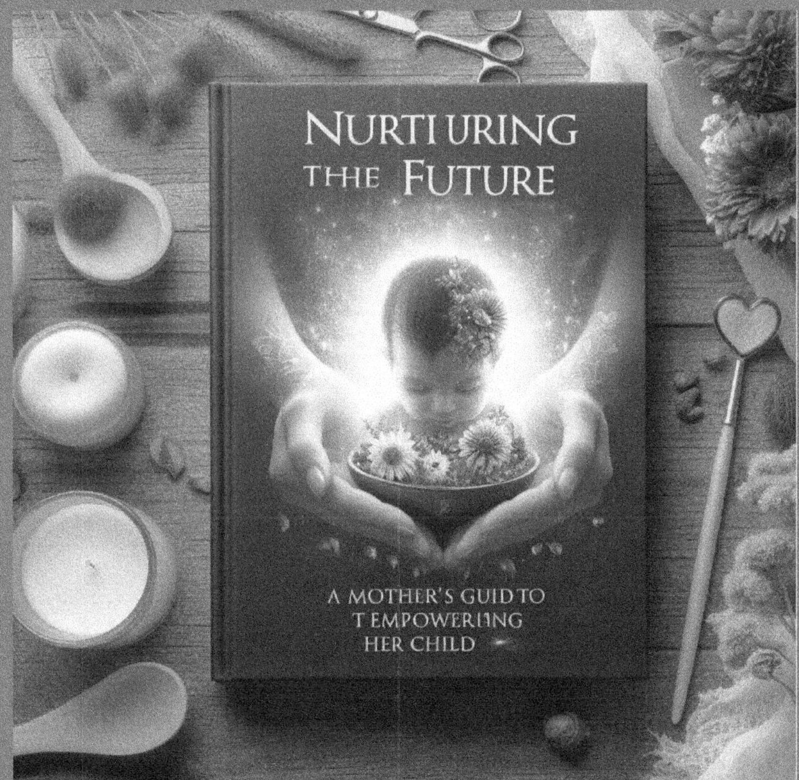

A Mother's Guide to Empowering Her Child

Table of Contents

Chapter 1: Introduction

- ➢ **The Significance Of Early Childhood Development**

- ➢ **Critical Period of Brain Development:**

- ➢ **Formation of Core Skills:**

- ➢ **Establishing Social and Emotional Competence:**

- ➢ **Impact on Health and Well-being:**

- ➢ **Reducing Achievement Gaps:**

- ➢ **Long-term Economic Benefits:**

The Significance Of Early Childhood Development

The significance of early childhood development is immense, as this critical period, typically spanning the first five years of a child's life, lays the groundwork for their future physical, cognitive, emotional, and social well-being. Physically, it's a time of rapid growth and development, necessitating proper nutrition, sufficient sleep, and regular health check-ups to ensure optimal growth. Activities promoting motor skills, like crawling and grasping, are vital. Cognitively, early childhood is characterized by profound brain development, with neural connections forming rapidly in response to stimuli. Engaging in activities such as reading and problem-solving is crucial for laying the foundation for future learning. Emotionally, children start forming their sense of self and learn emotional regulation through positive interactions and a nurturing environment. Socially, early childhood is when children learn to interact with others and navigate social norms, crucial for developing social skills and empathy. Overall, investing in early childhood development not only benefits individual children but also contributes to societal well-being by fostering future generations' potential and socio-economic development.

Critical Period of Brain Development

The critical period of brain development, typically spanning from prenatal stages through early childhood, represents a pivotal phase in a person's life. During this time, the brain undergoes rapid growth and forms crucial neural connections that lay the foundation for future cognitive functioning. This period is characterized by heightened neuroplasticity, meaning the brain is highly responsive to environmental stimuli and experiences, shaping its structure and function. The significance of the critical period of brain development cannot be overstated, as it sets the stage for various cognitive abilities such as language acquisition, sensory processing, and higher-order thinking skills. Exposure to enriching environments, nurturing relationships, and stimulating activities during this period can greatly enhance brain development and optimize cognitive outcomes. Conversely, adverse experiences or lack of stimulation during this critical window may lead to long-term deficits in cognitive functioning and neural connectivity. Understanding and prioritizing the critical period of brain development is essential for promoting optimal cognitive development and maximizing individual potential. By providing supportive environments, early interventions, and targeted interventions during this sensitive period, we can help ensure that children have the best possible start in life and lay a solid foundation for their future learning, behavior, and overall well-being.

Formation of Core Skills

The formation of core skills is a fundamental process that begins early in life and continues throughout one's development. These core skills encompass a wide range of abilities, including cognitive, social, emotional, and physical competencies, that are essential for navigating daily life and achieving success in various contexts. During the early years, the formation of core skills is particularly critical as the brain undergoes rapid growth and development. This period, often referred to as the critical window, is characterized by heightened neuroplasticity, allowing for the establishment of foundational skills such as language acquisition, problem-solving, emotional regulation, and social interaction. As children grow and mature, the formation of core skills becomes increasingly influenced by both genetics and environmental factors. Positive experiences, supportive relationships, and opportunities for exploration and learning play crucial roles in shaping and refining these skills over time. By recognizing the importance of early intervention and providing enriching environments, we can support the development of core skills and empower individuals to reach their full potential across the lifespan.

Establishing Social and Emotional Competence

Establishing social and emotional competence is essential for individuals to navigate interpersonal relationships, regulate their emotions, and adapt to various social situations effectively. This process begins in early childhood and continues throughout life, influenced by both genetic predispositions and environmental experiences. During the formative years, children learn to recognize and express their emotions, understand the feelings of others, and develop empathy and compassion. Positive interactions with caregivers, peers, and educators play a crucial role in shaping these social and emotional skills. Through play, communication, and modeling, children gradually acquire the necessary tools to navigate social interactions and manage their emotions appropriately. As individuals progress into adolescence and adulthood, the establishment of social and emotional competence becomes increasingly important for success in personal, academic, and professional domains. Strong social and emotional skills enable individuals to build meaningful relationships, communicate effectively, and navigate challenges and conflicts constructively. By fostering a supportive environment and providing opportunities for social and emotional learning, we can empower individuals to develop the competence needed to thrive in all aspects of life.

Impact on Health and Well-being

The impact of social and emotional competence on health and well-being is profound, influencing various aspects of individuals' lives. Research indicates that individuals with strong social connections and effective emotional regulation skills tend to experience better physical health outcomes, including lower rates of chronic diseases and mortality. Furthermore, social and emotional competence plays a significant role in mental health and psychological well-being. Individuals who possess strong interpersonal skills and emotional resilience are better equipped to cope with stress, adversity, and life challenges. They are also more likely to experience higher levels of life satisfaction, happiness, and overall psychological well-being. Moreover, social and emotional competence is closely linked to positive social outcomes, such as increased social support, better relationship quality, and higher levels of community engagement. Strong social connections and effective communication skills contribute to a sense of belonging and fulfillment, fostering a supportive environment that promotes overall health and well-being for individuals and communities alike.

Reducing Achievement Gap

Reducing the achievement gap is a crucial goal in education, aiming to ensure that all students, regardless of background or circumstance, have equal opportunities to succeed academically. This gap refers to the disparities in educational outcomes between different groups of students, often along lines of race, socioeconomic status, and access to resources. Addressing the achievement gap requires a multifaceted approach that encompasses various factors contributing to educational inequality. This includes addressing systemic barriers, providing equitable access to quality education, implementing culturally responsive teaching practices, and offering targeted interventions to support students who are at risk of falling behind. By narrowing the achievement gap, we can create a more inclusive and equitable educational system that empowers all students to reach their full potential. This not only benefits individual students by improving their academic outcomes and future opportunities but also fosters a more just and equitable society where every individual has the chance to thrive.

Long-term Economic Benefits

Investing in education yields long-term economic benefits that extend far beyond the classroom. A well-educated workforce is crucial for driving innovation, increasing productivity, and fostering economic growth in both local and global economies. By providing individuals with access to quality education and equipping them with the skills and knowledge needed to succeed in the workforce, we can create a more competitive and resilient economy. Furthermore, education plays a key role in reducing income inequality and promoting social mobility. Individuals with higher levels of education typically earn higher wages and are more likely to secure stable employment opportunities. This not only improves their own economic well-being but also contributes to overall economic prosperity by increasing consumer spending, tax revenues, and economic stability. Moreover, investing in education generates positive externalities that benefit society as a whole. A more educated population is associated with lower crime rates, improved health outcomes, and increased civic engagement. These social benefits contribute to a healthier, safer, and more cohesive society, laying the groundwork for sustained economic growth and prosperity in the long term.

Chapter2:   Building   a   Strong Foundation

"Building a Strong Foundation to Empower Her Child" is a comprehensive guide that delves into the essentia principles and practices mothers can employ to foster their child's growth, confidence, and resilience. This topic is centered around the pivotal role mothers play in laying the groundwork for their child's future success and well-being.At its core, this guide emphasizes the importance of nurturing a supportive and empowering environment for children. It explores various aspects of parenting, including emotional support, cognitive development, and social skills building, to help mothers create a strong foundation for their child's growth and development.Within this guide, mothers are provided with practical strategies and insights for instilling a positive mindset, fostering independence, and nurturing their child's unique strengths and talents. It underscores the significance of open communication, active listening, and empathy in building strong parent-child relationships and fostering a sense of trust and security.

Empowerment is a central theme of this guide, as mothers are encouraged to empower their children to take ownership of their actions, make informed decisions, and navigate life's challenges with confidence. It emphasizes the importance of teaching resilience, problem-solving skills, and emotional intelligence, equipping children with the tools they need to thrive in an ever-changing world.Furthermore, this guide recognizes the importance of self-care for mothers, highlighting the need to prioritize their own well-being in order to better support their children effectively. It encourages mothers to cultivate a balance between nurturing their child's growth and maintaining their own personal fulfillment and identity.

Overall, "Building a Strong Foundation to Empower Her Child" serves as a roadmap for mothers to navigate the journey of parenthood with intentionality, compassion, and purpose. It empowers mothers to create a nurturing and empowering environment that enables their children to reach their full potential and become confident, resilient, and empowered individuals.

Chapter 3: Cultivating a Growth Mindset

"Cultivating a Growth Mindset to Empower Her Child" is a dynamic exploration into the transformative power of adopting a growth mindset in nurturing children towards success and fulfillment. This topic underscores the critical role parents, particularly mothers, play in shaping their child's attitudes towards learning, resilience, and personal development.At its core, this guide encourages mothers to embrace and promote the concept of a growth mindset, which champions the belief that intelligence, abilities, and talents can be developed through dedication, effort, and resilience. Unlike a fixed mindset, which views abilities as innate and unchangeable, a growth mindset fosters a sense of optimism, perseverance, and a willingness to embrace challenges as opportunities for growth.

Within this guide, mothers are provided with practical strategies and insights for instilling a growth mindset in their children. It emphasizes the importance of praising effort, persistence, and resilience, rather than focusing solely on outcomes or innate abilities. By fostering a culture of learning, curiosity, and self-improvement, mothers can empower their children to embrace challenges, learn from failures, and cultivate a lifelong love of learning. Furthermore, this guide explores the role of language and feedback in shaping children's mindset and self-perception. It encourages mothers to use language that promotes effort, progress, and the value of mistakes as learning opportunities. By providing constructive feedback and reframing setbacks as part of the learning process, mothers can help their children develop resilience and a positive attitude towards overcoming obstacles.

Empowerment is a central theme of this guide, as mothers are encouraged to model a growth mindset in their own attitudes and behaviors. By demonstrating a willingness to learn, adapt, and persevere in the face of challenges, mothers can inspire their children to cultivate similar qualities and embrace their full potential.Ultimately, "Cultivating a Growth Mindset to Empower Her Child" serves as a roadmap for mothers to foster a culture of growth, resilience, and self-belief in their children. It empowers mothers to nurture their children's innate potential and equip them with the mindset and skills needed to thrive in an ever-changing world.

Chapter 4: Encouraging Academic Success

"Encouraging Academic Success to Empower Her Child" is a comprehensive guide that explores the strategies and approaches mothers can utilize to support their child's academic journey and empower them to achieve their full potential in education. This topic emphasizes the critical role mothers play in fostering a positive attitude towards learning, academic achievement, and personal growth.At its core, this guide encourages mothers to create a supportive and nurturing environment that prioritizes education and academic success. It emphasizes the importance of setting high expectations, providing encouragement, and offering practical support to help children excel academically.

Within this guide, mothers are provided with practical strategies and insights for promoting academic success. It delves into the importance of establishing routines, creating a conducive study environment, and setting achievable goals to help children stay focused and motivated in their academic pursuits. Furthermore, this guide explores the role of parental involvement in education and highlights the various ways mothers can actively support their child's learning journey. From monitoring academic progress to providing assistance with homework and assignments, mothers are empowered to play an active role in their child's education and academic development.

Empowerment is a central theme of this guide, as mothers are encouraged to instill confidence, resilience, and a growth mindset in their children. By celebrating achievements, offering constructive feedback, and encouraging perseverance in the face of challenges, mothers can help their children develop the skills and mindset needed to succeed academically and beyond.Moreover, this guide recognizes the importance of fostering a love of learning and curiosity in children. It encourages mothers to nurture their child's interests, expose them to diverse learning opportunities, and instill a lifelong passion for education. Ultimately, "Encouraging Academic Success to Empower Her Child" serves as a roadmap for mothers to support and empower their children in their academic endeavors. By providing guidance, encouragement, and practical support, mothers can help their children unlock their full potential and achieve academic success, paving the way for a bright and promising future.

Chapter 5: Fostering Emotional Intelligence

"Fostering Emotional Intelligence to Empower Her Child" is a comprehensive guide designed to equip mothers with the tools and strategies to nurture their child's emotional intelligence, thereby empowering them to navigate life's challenges with resilience, empathy, and self-awareness. This topic recognizes the crucial role mothers play in helping their children develop emotional intelligence, which is essential for building strong relationships, managing stress, and making sound decisions. At its core, this guide emphasizes the importance of fostering a supportive and emotionally nurturing environment in the home. Mothers are encouraged to cultivate open communication channels, where children feel safe expressing their feelings and thoughts without fear of judgment. By validating and acknowledging their child's emotions, mothers can help them develop a deeper understanding of their own feelings and those of others.

Within this guide, mothers are provided with practical strategies and insights for promoting emotional intelligence in their children. It delves into the importance of teaching children to identify and label their emotions, as well as to regulate them effectively. Through activities such as storytelling, role-playing, and problem-solving, mothers can help their children develop crucial emotional management skills.Furthermore, this guide explores the role of empathy and perspective-taking in nurturing emotional intelligence. Mothers are encouraged to model empathy in their interactions with others and to teach their children the importance of considering different viewpoints and experiences. By fostering empathy, mothers can help their children build strong interpersonal relationships and navigate social situations with grace and understanding.

Empowerment is a central theme of this guide, as mothers are encouraged to empower their children to become active participants in their emotional growth and development. By teaching them coping strategies, problem-solving skills, and resilience-building techniques, mothers can help their children cultivate the emotional resilience needed to thrive in today's complex world. Moreover, this guide recognizes the importance of self-care for mothers in their role as emotional mentors. It emphasizes the need for mothers to prioritize their own well-being, so they can effectively support and nurture their children's emotional intelligence. Ultimately, "Fostering Emotional Intelligence to Empower Her Child" serves as a roadmap for mothers to cultivate a nurturing and emotionally intelligent environment in which their children can thrive. By providing guidance, support, and practical tools, mothers can empower their children to develop the emotional intelligence needed to lead fulfilling and successful lives.

Chapter 6: Nurturing Talents and Passions

"Chapter 6: Nurturing Talents and Passions to Empower Her Child" is a dynamic exploration into the ways mothers can identify, nurture, and support their child's unique talents and passions, thereby empowering them to pursue their interests with confidence and enthusiasm. This chapter recognizes the importance of fostering a supportive and encouraging environment where children feel empowered to explore their interests, develop their talents, and pursue their passions to their fullest potential.

At its core, this chapter emphasizes the significance of recognizing and celebrating the diverse talents and passions that children possess. Mothers are encouraged to observe their child's interests, strengths, and natural inclinations, and to provide opportunities for them to explore and develop these areas further. Within this chapter, mothers are provided with practical strategies and insights for nurturing their child's talents and passions. It delves into the importance of providing a supportive and encouraging environment where children feel free to express themselves creatively and pursue their interests with enthusiasm. From enrolling them in extracurricular activities to providing access to resources and mentors, mothers are empowered to create opportunities for their children to cultivate their talents and passions. Furthermore, this chapter explores the role of encouragement and positive reinforcement in nurturing talents and passions. Mothers are encouraged to praise their child's efforts and achievements, and to provide constructive feedback and guidance to help them grow and improve in their chosen pursuits.

Empowerment is a central theme of this chapter, as mothers are encouraged to empower their children to pursue their passions with confidence and determination. By instilling a sense of self-belief and resilience, mothers can help their children overcome obstacles and setbacks on their journey to realizing their full potential. Moreover, this chapter recognizes the importance of fostering a growth mindset in children, wherein they view challenges as opportunities for learning and growth. By teaching children to embrace failure as a natural part of the learning process and to persevere in the face of adversity, mothers can help them develop the resilience and determination needed to succeed in their chosen endeavors. Ultimately, "Chapter 6: Nurturing Talents and Passions to Empower Her Child" serves as a valuable resource for mothers seeking to support and encourage their child's journey of self-discovery and personal development. By providing guidance, support, and encouragement, mothers can empower their children to pursue their passions with confidence, enthusiasm, and a sense of purpose.

Chapter 7: Setting Goals and Planning for the Future

"Setting Goals and Planning for the Future to Empower Her Child" is an insightful exploration into the vital role mothers play in guiding their children to set meaningful goals, develop action plans, and navigate the path towards a fulfilling and successful future. This topic recognizes the importance of instilling a sense of purpose, direction, and agency in children from a young age, empowering them to take ownership of their aspirations and work towards achieving them. At its core, this topic emphasizes the significance of goal-setting as a powerful tool for personal growth and achievement. Mothers are encouraged to engage their children in conversations about their dreams, interests, and aspirations, and to help them identify specific, achievable goals that align with their values and passions. Within this exploration, mothers are provided with practical strategies and insights for guiding their children through the goal-setting process. It delves into the importance of setting SMART (Specific, Measurable, Achievable, Relevant, Time-bound) goals, breaking them down into manageable steps, and developing action plans to turn aspirations into reality.

Furthermore, this topic explores the role of vision and visualization in goal-setting and planning for the future. Mothers are encouraged to help their children envision their desired outcomes, visualize success, and cultivate a positive mindset that fuels motivation and resilience in the face of challenges. Empowerment is a central theme of this exploration, as mothers are encouraged to empower their children to take ownership of their goals and aspirations. By providing support, encouragement, and guidance, mothers can help their children develop the self-discipline, perseverance, and resilience needed to pursue their goals with determination and confidence. Moreover, this topic recognizes the importance of adaptability and flexibility in goal-setting and planning for the future.

Mothers are encouraged to teach their children the value of embracing change, learning from setbacks, and adjusting their plans as needed to stay on course towards their desired outcomes. Ultimately, "Setting Goals and Planning for the Future to Empower Her Child" serves as a valuable resource for mothers seeking to empower their children to take control of their destinies and create a future filled with purpose, fulfillment, and success. By providing guidance, support, and encouragement, mothers can help their children navigate the journey of goal-setting and planning with confidence, resilience, and a sense of possibility.

Chapter 8: Embracing Challenges and Overcoming Obstacles

"Embracing Challenges and Overcoming Obstacles to Empower Her Child" is an insightful exploration into the transformative power of resilience, perseverance, and adaptability in helping children thrive in the face of adversity. This topic acknowledges the inevitability of challenges and obstacles in life and underscores the critical role mothers play in equipping their children with the skills and mindset needed to overcome them. At its core, this exploration emphasizes the importance of reframing challenges as opportunities for growth and learning. Mothers are encouraged to foster a growth mindset in their children, wherein setbacks and obstacles are viewed as temporary hurdles rather than insurmountable barriers. By teaching children to embrace challenges with courage and determination, mothers empower them to develop resilience and resourcefulness in navigating life's ups and downs.

Within this exploration, mothers are provided with practical strategies and insights for helping their children embrace challenges and overcome obstacles. It delves into the importance of teaching children problem-solving skills, coping mechanisms, and stress-management techniques to navigate difficult situations effectively. Furthermore, this topic explores the role of perseverance and tenacity in overcoming obstacles. Mothers are encouraged to model perseverance in their own attitudes and behaviors, demonstrating resilience in the face of adversity and showing their children that setbacks are an inherent part of the learning process. Empowerment is a central theme of this exploration, as mothers are encouraged to empower their children to take an active role in overcoming challenges. By providing support, encouragement, and guidance, mothers can help their children develop the confidence and self-efficacy needed to tackle obstacles head-on and emerge stronger on the other side. Moreover, this exploration recognizes the importance of fostering a supportive and nurturing environment where children feel safe to take risks and make mistakes. Mothers are encouraged to provide unconditional love and encouragement, creating a space where children feel empowered to experiment, learn, and grow. Ultimately, "Embracing Challenges and Overcoming Obstacles to Empower Her Child" serves as a valuable resource for mothers seeking to instill resilience, perseverance, and adaptability in their children. By providing guidance, support, and encouragement, mothers can help their children navigate life's challenges with confidence, courage, and a sense of possibility.!!

REFRENCE

Bandura, A. (1977). Self-efficacy: Toward a unifying theory of behavioral change. Psychological Review, 84(2), 191–215.

Dweck, C. S. (2006). Mindset: The new psychology of success. Random House.

Goleman, D. (1995). Emotional intelligence: Why it can matter more than IQ. Bantam Books.

Gottman, J. M., & DeClaire, J. (1997). Raising an emotionally intelligent child: The heart of parenting. Simon and Schuster.

Kabat-Zinn, J. (1994). Wherever you go, there you are: Mindfulness meditation in everyday life. Hyperion.

Siegel, D. J., & Bryson, T. P. (2012). The whole-brain child: 12 revolutionary strategies to nurture your child's developing mind. Delacorte Press.

Pink, D. H. (2009). Drive: The surprising truth about what motivates us. Riverhead Books.

Rosen, L. D., & Lim, A. F. (2011). Media and technology use predicts ill-being among children, preteens and teenagers independent of the negative health impacts of exercise and eating habits. Computers in Human Behavior, 29(5), 2161–2170.

Seligman, M. E. P. (2011). Flourish: A visionary new understanding of happiness and well-being. Free Press.

Siegel, D. J. (2013). Brainstorm: The power and purpose of the teenage brain. Penguin Group.

Weissbourd, R. (2009). The parents we mean to be: How well-intentioned adults undermine children's moral and emotional development. Houghton Mifflin Harcourt.

GOOD LUCK

9 798325 360312